Sending Mama To Her Room

Seven Locks Press
P.O. Box 25689
Santa Ana, CA 92799
800-354-5348

Individual Sales. This book is available through most bookstores or can be ordered directly from Seven Locks Press at the above address.

Quantity Sales. Special discounts are available on quantity purchases by corporations, associations, and others. For details, contact the "Special Sales Department" at the publisher's address above.

Printed in the United States of America

Library of Congress Cataloging-in-Publication Data is available from the publisher.

ISBN 1-931643-19-9

Cover design by
Sparrow Advertising & Design

Table of Contents

Preface

The best thing happens when you tell people what you are writing a book about. They share their stories with you and they share names of other people who have stories. They e-mail you pieces they think would be great in the book. ***And, most of all, they tell you how very much they wish you had written the book when they needed it.***

This book contains real stories and imaginary ones (based on real experiences) about taking care of "mama." The seeds for this book come from the eighteen years my mother and I lived together. I was her primary caregiver, raising two children as a single parent, while careening through the corporate fast track–suddenly exit-ramping into unemployed–then climbing onto the woman business owner roller coaster <u>and</u> juggling health problems <u>and</u> exploring several significant/semi-significant/non-significant personal relationships, as well as all those other out-of-the-blue curve balls life throws you. These seeds have been fertilized by my imagination, watered by the input of so many wonderful people (whom I will not list, but they know who they are) and have grown into this book.

If you are a caregiver, what I am hoping you will harvest from this bumper crop of stories, anecdotes, poems, sayings *et al* is some comfort, an understanding that you are not alone in your feelings and frustrations, that there is support out there for you and that you will, indeed, run the gamut of emotions as you care for that loved one. My goal is that you will get a feeling of hope from this book, see that you are not alone, and that the emotion you will express most is laughter. I learned many, many things from being a caregiver, but the most important was that she (or he) who laughs, lasts.

If you are not currently a caregiver and are under the age of sixty, the odds are that you will become one. If you are a member of the Baby Boomer generation, you undoubtedly have already heard that you will be caring for a parent for as many years, if not more, than you have spent raising your children. (And if your children were like mine and hung around the house until well into their twenties, many of those years will overlap.) If you are in the thirty-something group, 95% of you will be caring for an aging loved one at some point.

Caregiving is not a passing fad. It is a phenomenon that is going to grow exponentially in the next twenty years. Most people are never truly prepared for it – physically, financially, emotionally, spiritually - and I am not talking about the aging person. I am talking about the caregiver and the caregiver's family, friends, co-workers, acquaintances, even total strangers. Being a caregiver affects everyone!

Last, but not least, I want to dedicate this book to all the people who were there for me during those times I wanted to send mama to her room. I love you all.

Let the Caregiving begin

I entered the arena of caregiving without knowing it in 1978, when my Dad died at the age of 64. I asked my Mom to live with me. We had never discussed it before then. In fact, we had never talked about the "what if's" of either of them growing old. Mom and Dad had been married for thirty-seven years. Although he had heart problems, he had a pacemaker and no one expected him to die. Least of all, me. I thought old age was being 80. The one we had worried about was Mom because she had so many health problems. I just didn't see how she could carry on by herself, so I asked her to live with me. It just felt right. She had always been there for me and now I was going to be there for her.

You have to understand, I have no *mommy dearest* stories. Mom had always been my confidante, support, guide and friend. I come by my sense of humor honestly. My favorite memories of growing up are the hours I would sit on the kitchen counter talking to her about my day at school, my friends and my feelings. One day when I went to lunch with Mom, she let me have my first cigarette. It was our secret because Dad would have had a fit because we both knew he would not approve. After all, he paid for the voice lessons - all those years of classical training - and would not have been at all happy about it. Of course, no one knew how harmful cigarettes were then, but being a doctor, his diagnosis would have been that I shouldn't do it because it "wasn't good for me."

My mom was special. She was my Scout leader, my dressmaker, and my super creative birthday party producer. I picked up my arts and crafts abilities from her. We played duets on the piano. We both loved Christmas and spending the whole year searching for the perfect gifts for everyone in the family. She showed me, through her close friendships, how to be a real friend. Once, when I was in junior high, she had an operation on her back. She was in bed for a long time and I became the Mom -- cooking, cleaning, taking care of her. It was fun and I was glad to do it.

Good times. Great memories. Even when I recalled those of taking care of her, I only remembered it as a good experience.

When we moved in together, we bought a unique housing arrangement that provided her with a little bungalow of her own and me with a three-bedroom house. The garage connected the units. She voluntarily "re-upped" for motherhood by helping me raise the kids. I worked. She was there for them when they came home from school. We thought alike; we sounded alike. The kids got it in stereo! They knew they couldn't play us against each other (although they tried). When they called home on the phone, they didn't know which one they were talking to. It was great. (At least I thought it was. I'm not sure how thrilled the kids were with having two mothers!)

Time passed. She replaced the cane with a walker, but still was very independent. We talked only occasionally about her growing older, but never had any serious discussions. I equated old age with gray hair and since she didn't have any, I dismissed it.

She contacted the family attorney, made a Living Will and set up power of attorney for me so that, when the time came, I could make sure that she could die with dignity without any heroic measures.

She told me what she had done and made me promise her that, "when the time came," I would not allow her to go on in pain and misery and that, if before then, she became a burden, I would "take the appropriate measures." I guaranteed her that if she ever got “like that” I would send her to her room. I meant it as a joke. We both laughed. For years, whenever she had a bad day, when her legs got weak or she was in a lot of pain, I would threaten to send her to her room. It became sort of a private joke between us. All the while, things were changing. She could do less and I did more.

I naively thought this was what taking care of your parent was all about. I didn't understand why so much was being written about it. Sure there were some tough times, but we are both strong people. We could handle it. All it took was making a joke about it.

We had always been able to find the light side of any tough time, but it got harder than either of us ever thought it would. There were more and more bad days. We moved a wheelchair into the house so she could get around while I was at work. More problems, more medicines. There were infections that caused her to lose all ability to even get out of bed. Each time we'd hang in there and she'd recover, but not exactly as great as she had been before. She hated depending on the kids and me for everything. After a while, she could no longer be left alone at all. We hired outside help to do things I could no longer handle alone, like lifting her.

These were not happy times. We both had lost our independence. It was very hard for Mom to maintain a feeling of worth when I was cooking her meals, helping her dress and doing many of the things she could no longer do. Her sense of dignity was really lost when I had to change her Depends.

My life had returned to the way it was when I had two small children. With one huge difference. We were not very good at any of this. She was not good at asking for help. I was not good at remembering what needed to be done. I was not even a very good wheelchair driver!

There were chipped paint marks along the walls and doors to prove it!

I was determined to work it out, however, and not grow to resent her in the process. I expected her to understand what I was going through because she had been through it.

When I was a teenager, both my mother's mother and my father's father lived with us. Maybe Mom had selective amnesia, but I remember both of them sitting at the dinner table bickering because they thought the other one had been given a bigger portion. And I can remember how they tried to get my parents to take sides just as my brother and I had done with them.

As with so many families, the day came when Mom could no longer physically take care of them and they had to be moved to nursing homes. Neither one of them adjusted well. My grandmother always thought her things were being stolen and that everyone was talking behind her back. My grandfather vowed he would die before my wedding day and he did. I have always believed he willed it.

Those memories haunted me. The real problem was I still wanted to believe that this was only temporary and that she would once again be able to completely take care of herself. But it didn't happen. What we needed to figure out - together - was how we were going to handle the rest of her life. However, like so many people, we talked around the issue and waited until there seemed to be no choices left and we had to do something. When that time came, neither one of us was truly prepared. She was angry and bitter that this was happening to her and I knew it was no longer a joke because I was actually sending my mother to her room.

Hindsight is always 20/20.

If I only knew then, what I know now. And this is what I know . . .

You never stop loving the person you are taking care of, but there are days when you don't like them very much.

Being a caregiver doesn't mean sacrificing your health - mental or physical.

While God did make it so only women can birth children, She never meant for caregiving to be a woman's sole responsibility.

An elder can be bribed to do something she doesn't want to do. Just threaten to withhold dessert.

There are many stages of caregiving-it goes from being relatively easy to being virtually impossible.

Never raise your voice in anger to an elder. Whisper your anger. Chances are, they won't hear you then.

Parenting a parent is not like raising children. When children talk back to us, we send them to their rooms. When parents talk back to us, we want to go to ours.

I learned more from my mother and about my mother during my years of caregiving than I ever knew when I was younger.

If I could do it over, there are many things I would do differently, but I would definitely do it again.

It's a Fact!

The older population will burgeon between the years 2010 and 2030 when the "baby boom" generation reaches age 65.

By 2030, there will be about 70 million older persons, more than twice their number in 2000. People 65+ represented 12.4% of the population in the year 2000 but is expected to grow to be 20% of the population by 2030.

As of 2001, women accounted for approximately 58% of the population age 60 and older and 50% of the population age 85 and older.

Women are the fastest growing segment of the older population.

The average life expectancy for women is 79 years.

7 out of 10 “baby boom” women will outlive their husbands.

The number of women ages 100 or older will double in the next 10 years.

Compared with men, older women are three times more likely to be living alone, spend more years and a larger percentage of their lifetime disabled, are nearly twice as likely to reside in a nursing home, and are more than twice as likely to live in poverty.

Administration on Aging
www.aoa.gov/factsheets

Carol stood in the doorway, watching her mother talk to the television.

"You ought to be ashamed of yourself!" her mother yelled. "Parading around there half-naked! Just wait until your father sees you, young lady. You won't be able to sit down for a month after he takes the strap to you."

Carol sat down beside her mother. "Mom, don't get so upset. It's only a TV show."

Her mother looked at her and raised her eyebrow. "Just who do you think you are, calling me Mom? Only my daughter can call me that and she's not here. I just saw her in that motion picture show. She was prancing around in a skimpy little dress, right there for God and everyone to see! So, who <u>are</u> you?"

Carol sat and stared at her mother, deciding how to answer. She glanced at the TV and saw the woman her mother had been talking to. Oh great, she thought, she thinks her daughter is Pamela Lee. So who does she think I am? And even more important, just who is this person in my mother's body?

"Mrs. White, I have known you for a long time, but it seems you don't remember me," Carol answered. "In fact, you're the very first person I ever met in my whole life!"

"That's nice, dear," her mother said, patting her hand. "Did you know my husband, Paul, too?"

"Oh, yes, he was the most wonderful man," Carol replied, and smiled at the memory.

"Harrumph! I remember you now. You're that woman across the street who is always flirting with him. If you think you're going to steal my husband, think again girly. Others have tried, but all have failed," she spit out. "I know how to keep him on his leash."

Carol was flabbergasted. She had never heard her mother talk about her father that way. Their marriage had always been perfect. Where was this coming from?

"I'm not trying to steal your husband," Carol replied, remembering the single woman across the street from their house and how kind her father had been to her, taking out her trash cans, shoveling her walk. Carol was sure there had never been anything more than that. "He is very kind and helps me out, but I've never even asked him to."

Carol had learned to talk to her mother as though she was a stranger. Over the past year her mother's mind had become so clouded that it was hard to tell when she was in the present and when she was in the past. She had learned to talk to her in the present tense though, because her mother would become very upset if Carol talked about her father or anyone else who had died, in the past tense.

"Oh, yes, he's always helping women out, a regular knight saving damsels in distress. But I'm his queen," her mother replied haughtily. "He told me it was silly for me to be jealous of his being nice to women.

"You know," she cackled wickedly, "he said I'm the only one who has access to the 'family jewels.' He had the 'jewels' and I had the money. So he isn't going to stray very far, girly."

Carol stared at her mother. Was this the woman her father was married to? This self-absorbed, caustic woman. The woman before her was not the wife and mother she remembered. But then again, her memories of the family were those from childhood. Her father had died when she was eighteen and her mother had become a gypsy of sorts, always traveling to strange and exotic places; then turning up periodically for short visits. She had lived this nomadic life for almost a quarter of a century, until she fell on the ice in London, hitting her head and suffering a severe concussion. Carol had flown over and sat by her bed for two months, thinking her mother would never wake up. But she did. And they flew back to the States and her mother moved in with her.

Only the woman who awakened was not her mother. Who was this woman, who had nasty things to say about everybody, seemed to have only sad, bitter memories and was totally self-centered? Where had her mother gone? Her mother, who always called her princess, who hugged her and made her feel so loved. Carol's mother turned away from the TV and called out, "Oh, papa, I am indeed your princess! Did you bring me the doll I want? Oh, goody. She's going to be my little girl and I'll be the queen and she can be the princess."

Then, turning to Carol, she reached out her hand and sighed, "Oh, there you are. Where have you been, princess? I know you're really busy, but I wish you'd visit me more often. Now, don't act like such a stranger. Give your mother a hug."

ADL's

What they don't tell you in any of the caregiving guides is that as your mother's ADL's (Activities of Daily Living) decline, yours go up! And it's not just the ADL's, it's also the IADL's (Instrumental Activities of Daily Living). Before anyone enters into caregiving, someone should warn them that the ratio of decline to increase is about 4:1. Let me explain:

ADL's include getting in and out of bed, bathing, dressing, eating, getting around inside, and using the toilet.

Mom's loss began simply by needing a little help getting her house organized and adapted so she could manage. We put up handrails, removed all the scatter rugs, cushioned the sharp corners of furniture and put all the essentials for her comfort - pillows, books, glasses, TV remote, tissues, telephone, playing cards, pens, paper, etc. on an end table next to her favorite chair. When the time came that she needed help getting in and out of bed, getting dressed and using the toilet, we moved her into our house.

We thought it would help all of us if we put a monitor in Mom's room so she could call us when she wanted or needed to get out of bed. What we soon came to realize was that Mom didn't sleep when we slept! Like a small child, she would take a nap in the afternoon, be ready for bed as soon as the news was over, but was ready to get up at 5:30 in the morning! With our kids when they were little, the early morning wake-up could be delayed by giving them a bottle or bringing them into bed with us, where they'd doze off again for at least another hour. Now, if you would like to see my husband shudder from head to toe, just ask him to envision bringing my mother into bed with us!

Getting dressed was another activity that made me think of my kids. Mom would change her mind half a dozen times about what she wanted to wear. Of course, she wouldn't change her mind until after I had struggled to get the shirts over her head (a real challenge since she couldn't raise her arms over her head), get her pants up, first while she sat in a chair and then as she held me in a headlock, terrified that she was going to fall while I pulled her pants up. (The Rock could have learned a few holds from my mother!) I tried to solve these problems by buying house dresses that were easy to get on her arms and had front snap closings. Of course, she hated them because she said they made her feel like an old woman and I didn't have the heart to point out the obvious to her.

I've got to tell you though that the real test of whether you're going to be able to handle caregiving is helping your mother go to the toilet. There is just no dignified, privacy-protected way to do this and it is uncomfortable and embarrassing for both. The same is true with bathing, but there comes a time when there are just no choices left and a caregiver's gotta do what a caregiver's gotta do. (If you think this is hard for mothers and daughters, let me tell you, it's still easier than mothers and sons. Just ask my brother!)

ADL's can double the workload, work off at least 200 calories a day, and leave the caregiver pretty darned pooped. Ah, but then there are the IADL's that make ADL's seem like really low impact aerobics.

IADL's included the ability to do heavy housework, laundry,

meal preparation, grocery shopping, getting around outside, getting to places outside of walking distance, money management, using the telephone, and taking medications.

Before she moved in with us, I would run over to Mom's and get her dinner because she could no longer reach things in the cupboard, lift the saucepan on the stove or carry a plate to the table. She needed more hands so she could keep hers on her walker for balance and steadiness. So I cooked her dinner first and then went home and cooked dinner for my family.

I did all her grocery shopping which invariably ended up in anger and frustration. I had her list, of course, but didn't have the crystal ball required to know what brands she preferred or what treats she had in her mind (which she hadn't written down) that I was supposed to know somehow. Chocolate was one of them, but it mattered not, even when I remembered because I never, I repeat never, bought the right chocolate. If I bought a candy bar, she wanted ice cream. If I bought chocolate-covered graham crackers, she wanted fudge bars. No wonder, I can't win the lottery. My powers of making the right choice are absolutely nil!

After Mom moved in with us, I realized that having her with us was just like having another kid. For a woman who didn't get out, she sure had a lot of laundry (and she ALWAYS left tissues in her pockets and I ALWAYS forgot to check). She would bicker with our kids about everything, especially which channel to watch and her time to use the phone.

And the music duel just about drove me crazy! Imagine, if you will, standing in the hall with the pounding of heavy metal "music" (and I use the word loosely) at full volume, assaulting you from one direction and the lovely, saccharine lyrics of Lawrence Welk's crew wafting at the top sound level from the other direction. Beats Chinese water torture, I'm here to tell you.

In fact, I think the only thing my kids had in common with their grandmother was that they were all going deaf.

And if you think sibling rivalry makes you want to send everyone to designated corners, it's nothing compared to the rivalry when a parent moves in.

For us, it came to a head when we got Mom her own phone. We had steadfastly refused to get the kids their own phone. If they wanted one, they had to pay for it and there were many heated arguments about their "right" to have a phone of their own.

To stop the fighting over the phone between Mom and the kids, we put one in her room and thought that would make life pleasant. That is, until the first bill came in and we discovered that Mom was letting the kids use her phone to make long distance calls, no less, as long as they "paid" for their calls by sneaking snacks into her room. No wonder her blood sugar level was sky high, let alone my blood pressure, when I discovered what was going on. I'm not proud of the resolution because we caved in and now we're on one of those family cell phone plans. I just hope the kids realize that they are spending their inheritance now by reaching out and touching all those friends of theirs.

Most people think that our parents lose their will to live when their driver's licenses are taken away from them. I think it happens when you have to take the checkbook away. As all children will tell you, their sense of independence starts with that coveted allowance and being able to hold it in their own hands and hide it in their own secret place. Our parents, when they get older, are the same way. Mom insisted on having a hundred dollars at all times - in singles. She doled them out to the kids to get them to turn down their music; to the neighbor's children to get them to buy candy for her which she hid under her underwear; to offer to the postman for ringing the doorbell to hand her a package; to tuck into envelopes to send off to feed children in other countries; to purchase hairnets from the mail order catalogue; or to include with her letters to government officials asking them to take her dollar and do something good, for once, for this wonderful country of ours.

When we first moved her in and my husband started going through her box of "important papers," he found bills that hadn't been paid and notices that hadn't been acknowledged. He also found a checkbook that hadn't been balanced in years. The weeks and weeks of getting that straightened out were clearly reflected in the increased spending on aspirin and antacid tablets.

Once you reach the IADL level, you should be good for at least a 400-calorie burn a day and total exhaustion by the end of each day. That is, unless, you are eating all the snacks you've taken from your Mom's underwear drawer.

Aw, God, Give Me a Break!

Hey, don't even get me started! You think you have it rough taking care of your mother. I'm taking care of my grandmother. And that's not the half of it. I'm doing it because my mother's pregnant! Wow, what a surprise that was. I thought Dad was going to have a heart attack. He thought her moodiness was PMS. She thought it was the change of life. Well, I'm here to tell you this whole thing has changed my life!

This is not my idea of how I'd be spending my teenage years. It's really freaked me out. No way am I going to have friends over to my house and see my own mother, waddling around, looking like she swallowed the biggest watermelon and hear my grandmother, yelling at the people on TV, just like she was talking to real people!

Mama couldn't really handle Grandma even before she got pregnant. Grandma's not sure where she is most days and she hasn't recognized me in ages. She thinks I'm my mother. So she's constantly yelling at me about my clothes, my hair, my make-up. If she had her way, I'd be wearing a white blouse, pleated skirt and Mary Jane's, with hose, of course. Right. And I wouldn't even talk unless someone spoke to me. Whatever.

This whole scene has ruined my life. I have to be up way before school in the morning to help Grandma get out of bed (she's down to 95 pounds, but it's hard to lift her out of bed because she's just like a really heavy sack of potatoes, you know.) She hates my being in the bathroom with her, helping her wash her face, putting her teeth in and going to the bathroom. (Hey, it's no fun for me either. She's got this loose, wrinkly skin all over. I mean all over, if you get my drift.) Meals aren't a picnic either. Most of the time, Grandma isn't really interested in the food and just bitches about how awful it tastes. Before I leave for school, I change her one last time and get her settled in her recliner chair with a clean, dry pad under her because she's always soaked before the agency aid comes in mid-morning to help her take a bath. The aid stays until I get home from school and then I take over. Lately, I've been cooking dinner too, because my mother's feet are so swollen she can't stand up long enough to get dinner.

My Dad says that all this is good practice for me for when I get married. I've gotta tell you, there's no way I'm EVER going to do all this stuff when I grow up. I mean once is enough, you know?

There are nights when I lie in bed and get really scared. Scared because I have this awful nightmare that this is never going to end. And then I have this really guilty feeling because, if it ends, it will mean that Grandma is dead.

It's not going to end after my mother has the baby either. I mean, jeez, she's almost forty. Taking care of a baby is going to take all her energy. I'll bet there will be times I'll be taking care of both my Grandma and the kid. It's just not fair. This isn't supposed to be my responsibility. I'm just a kid. I should be out having fun, dating that guy in my English class who keeps sending me signals.

You know what scares me the most? That I'll graduate from high school in three years and will have missed it all. When I'm old like Grandma, I won't have all those memories she has of when she was my age. I mean I know she has them because every time she talks it always starts with "When I was your age . . . "

Fact is, Grandma must have been amazing when she was my age. She was really pretty and "had to beat the boys off with a stick." There was one boy, George, who just wouldn't give up and, when she was eighteen she married him. That was my Grandpa, but I never knew him. He died when I was just a little kid.

Anyway, Grandma raised four kids and took in laundry to help out with the money. She did all kinds of things at school and at church and was real involved. My mother says she had loads and loads of friends, but most of them are dead or gone away now. I know she misses my Grandpa because she gets tears when she talks about him. Other than that, I'm not sure most of the time whether she's sad or not. Most of the time, she's not really here, not like in the today here. She's somewhere in the past. Maybe that's how you deal with getting old; you just stay in the past, in the "good old days."

Come on God, give me a break. I just can't believe that these are going to be my good old days!

PB&J . . .

When we are growing up, we never envision our parents being old. As adults, especially if we are lucky enough to live nearby, they don't even seem to change that much over the years. Until you wake up one morning and it has happened. Some alien has settled into your parents' bodies. This *being* walks more slowly and isn't sure-footed, has a mind that seems stuck in a time warp, remembering only those times you know about from family photographs, and is opinionated, forgetful, impatient and down-right cranky.

This person who used to adore your children when they were small and spoil them rotten and had the patience of Job with them, now is convinced that you have obviously failed as a parent because you aren't doing it the way they would. They "tsk, tsk, tsk" as you allow them to do things you were never allowed to do as a kid. Never mind that your kids' world is nothing like yours was as a child. But try to explain it? Forget it!

So here we are - stuck between the two - the peanut butter in the PB&J sandwich generation, holding it all together! Not me, you say. Want to bet? I'm here to tell you, it's going to happen.

I honestly believed my kids would grow up, graduate from college, begin their careers, find significant others and live elsewhere. I was sure that the day would come when I could walk into the living room and not find empty soft drink cans on the coffee table. It was going to work out great. My husband and I would have the place to ourselves. Ah, the age of innocence. It came to an end very quickly.

It all started with a broken hip. When my husband's mother fell it wasn't spectacular. In fact, she just stood up and fell down. The man who washes her windows found her. Since my husband was out of town on a business trip, they called me on the car phone and I got to her home just in time to see her being put into the ambulance. We assured each other that everything would be ok. But it wasn't that easy.

Mother didn't mend as well as the doctors had hoped. They said she should go to a nursing home to convalesce and get the physical therapy she needed. I visited her every day at lunch and after work. We had always gotten on well and had the same strange sense of humor (a fact her son thought just ran in the family until he started dating me). Our daily repartee kept her spirits up and, I think, became the daily entertainment for the entire staff at the nursing home. Until one day . . .

Mother was having a particularly uncomfortable day and was having a hissy fit because I came to visit her more than her son did. I offered to put her out of her misery. I was quickly ushered into the administrator's office, probably in preparation for calling the authorities. I was able to convince them that it was our way of dealing with the situation. From then on, they saw us as a strange, but harmless improv comedy team!

She put up with being in the nursing home for about two weeks and then she insisted on coming to our house because everyone there was "old." She could tell because they couldn't dress themselves, get their own meals, or take care of their own needs. And by comparison to Mother, they were. So we brought her to our house.

We turned our downstairs family room into her space. I ran the stairs, did the chores that were too difficult for her and helped her focus on more important things like seeing who could find the most pieces to finish the jigsaw puzzle, solve the mystery on TV or get the answer to the questions on *Jeopardy*. And so it went. She progressed to a walker and was talking about returning to her home. Until one day, when she tried to stand up and couldn't bear weight on her legs. Tests, hospitalization, and more tests. Therapy, tests, and more tests. No cure. Just adapt. But what did that mean?

It meant that the family room became Mother's. It meant there were more things she couldn't do for herself - showering, washing her hair, dressing, getting her meals, moving from her bed to a chair, going to the bathroom. I told my husband that we'd work it out because the alternative, looking into a nursing home, was something he couldn't even talk about, let alone consider.

I'm here to tell you, having your mother-in-law with you 24/7 must be God's idea of a really bad joke. Here I was taking care of her, waiting on her hand and foot, and what was she doing? Vying with me for my husband's attention! As soon as he came home from work, she wanted him to come sit with her and tell her how his day had been. She monopolized the conversation at dinner and after dinner came up with all kinds of "serious conversations" that she just had to have, in private, with him.

By the time we'd go to bed, he was exhausted, not only from his day at work, but also from having to be fully attentive to his mother. He'd lie in bed and complain, "I never have anytime to myself anymore! She wants my every waking moment spent with her! It's driving me crazy!"

Of course, if I started to complain, he would get upset with <u>me</u>. "She can't do those things herself. She doesn't like having to ask you to do them. In fact, she's always telling me how she hates to be a burden to you and what an angel you are for taking care of her."

Ok, I told myself, it could always be worse. Of course, I couldn't see how, but then, one cold January day, I got enrolled in *Real World 101*. Mother had a cold and was being even more demanding than normal. As I was running the stairs for the umpteenth time, I heard the garage door go up and the kitchen door open. Since it was the middle of the day, I was unsure who it was. I walked into the kitchen and there stood our daughter, with tears streaming down her face, and our two grandchildren, both of whom had runny noses. Oh great, I thought. Just what I need – visitors – with colds, no less!

"Mom, I've left Harold and the kids and I are moving back home."

Ok, God, enough's enough. Go test someone else for a while.

It's been six months now. Mother's still downstairs. Our daughter and grandchildren have taken over the upstairs. My husband and I are sleeping on the hide-a-bed couch in his den. At least they are all asleep and it's quiet. And I'm here in the kitchen, making the children's lunches for tomorrow. Yep, here I am, in the Sandwich Generation, and just like this peanut butter, I'm stuck in the middle.

After a while

After a while you learn

the subtle difference between

holding a hand and chaining a soul

and you learn

that love doesn't mean leaning

and company doesn't always mean security.

And you begin to learn

that kisses aren't contracts

and presents aren't promises

and you begin to accept your defeats

with your head up and your eyes ahead

with the grace of woman, not the grief of a child

and you learn

to build all your roads on today

because tomorrow's ground is

too uncertain for plans

and futures have a way of falling down

in mid-flight.

After a while you learn

that even sunshine burns

if you get too much

so you plant your own garden

and decorate your own soul

instead of waiting for someone

to bring you flowers.

And you learn that you really can endure

you really are strong

you really do have worth

and you learn

and you learn

with every goodbye, you learn...

Veronica A. Shoffstall wrote this verse while in college and yet its message is a powerful poem of the "coming of age" that happens to every woman when she assumes the role of being the caregiver.

I Wish I Had...

* Learned more about Mama's life and family because now there is no one to tell the stories

* Created more family times with my Mama and her grandchildren because her grandchildren made her feel young

* Asked for help sooner and not been so driven to try to do it all myself

* Understood better what it meant to Mama when we had to take away her driver's license, tell her she could no longer live alone and finally do all those simple things of daily living for her that we take for granted

* Known about the different insurance coverages that could have protected us financially

* Spent less time lugging Mama from her bed to her wheelchair and more time hugging her

* Told Mama how much I loved her, even those times when I didn't like her very much!

Deja Vu

Darla stood in the doorway watching her mother brush her granddaughter's hair. She noticed it was an obviously painful chore, trying to hold the brush with one arthritic hand and keep the squirming child still with the other.

"Darla, sit still!" the woman admonished.

"Gramma, I'm not Darla, I'm Amy. You always think I'm Mama," the child scolded.

"Why you're my precious little girl, that's what you are," Gramma said. "You are the cutest, smartest little girl in the world. And you are also the wiggliest!"

The child giggled. This hair brushing routine had been going on for four years now, ever since her gramma moved in with them. Mama said it was because Gramma was lonely and needed to be with her family. Amy suspected, being a very smart eight year old, that it was because Gramma wanted to pretend that she was young again and not so old and wrinkled and forgetful. But that was ok, because when she sat on Gramma's lap, Gramma would tell her stories about when Mama was a little girl and about Grandpa, who died when Amy was only four.

"Gramma, tell me the story again about how you and Grandpa met," Amy pleaded. It was her favorite story of all.

"Well, he tricked me into it, he did," she chuckled, as she continued to slowly brush her granddaughter's hair.

"When I was twelve, my Mama and Papa brought us to this country so we could live in a place where we were free, where we could *choose* the way we would live our lives," she began, always saying the word *choose* with great emphasis.

"We lived in a tiny little apartment, not much bigger than this room. It was over the grocery store where Mama and I went to do our daily shopping," she continued. "Each day, as the grocer was putting the groceries in Mama's sack, he would tell her that she could pay him then or pay him later. She always shook her head and handed him the money for the groceries.

"'Remember,' she would say, as we climbed the stairs with our food, 'you must always pay now because if you don't, the cost later on will be a price you pay a lifetime.'" Gramma always recited her mother's words reverently, as being one of the great truths in life.

"When I was in high school, Mama used to give me the list and I would go to the grocery store because Mama couldn't do the stairs anymore," she said, sighing at the recollection of her mother, sitting in the kitchen, trying so hard to peel the potatoes with her arthritic hands.

"The grocer's son would carry the groceries upstairs for me and then tell Mama the same thing, his father always said, 'You can pay me now or you can pay me later.' Mama just shook her head and struggled to get the money out of her coin purse to pay him.

"After I graduated from high school, I went to work at the perfume counter at Woolworth's, but lived at home to help Mama take care of my father and my little brother. That's what good daughter's do, Darla, they take care of their Mama," Gramma said, tapping the child on the arm with the hairbrush for emphasis.

"Anyway, when Mama died suddenly, I just continued on, taking care of my Papa and my little brother. Then Papa lost his job and we had no money. One day the grocer's son knocked on our door and, when I answered it, handed me a sack of groceries. 'I can't pay for these' I told him.

"'That's ok,' he said, smiling at me in the lovely way he always did. 'You can pay me later.'

"Now, I heard Mama's voice reprimanding me for accepting these groceries, when I couldn't pay for them, but I was scared because there was no money and I thought we would starve the way so many people had in the old country. So I accepted and accepted and accepted," she said contritely.

"One day I asked him what we owed him and, when he told me, I was so shocked I almost fainted! "We were never, ever going to be able to pay him and I was so ashamed that I hadn't heeded Mama's words."

She stopped and fumbled for the tissue that was always in her pocket. Amy wiggled around to help her get it out and watched while the old woman dabbed at her eyes.

“Then that grocer’s son took my hand and told me that he had paid his father each time he brought the groceries up out of his own money and that we didn’t owe him anything.

“Of course, I realized that my debt was now with this man and all of a sudden I was very afraid. After all, I was only nineteen and he was twenty-four. What had he done it for? How did he expect me to repay him? I looked into his sweet face and into those large, brown eyes and began to cry. And he just sat there, watching me.

“Well, actually he wasn’t just sitting there watching me. I looked down and he was holding my hand! Well, Lord, that made me cry even harder! I cried so hard I began to hiccup,” she giggled now, right along with her granddaughter.

“He got up and got me a glass of water,” she continued. “As I was drinking that water, I looked over that glass, saw the love in his eyes, and realized that I was going to be paying this bill the rest of my life," she concluded.

"Gramma, what did Grandpa always tell everyone," Amy urged, because she knew that the best part was still to come, the part where, when Gramma said it, she got the most wonderful smile on her face and just seemed to be so happy.

"Oh, he always said, buying those groceries was the best investment he ever made!"

Darla stood in the doorway and smiled. It was like looking back in time. How often had she sat on her Mama's lap, getting her hair brushed, and heard that story? And then at the end, Papa would look over his paper at her mother, smile at her and say, "Best investment I ever made!" Now she smiled, watching her daughter and her mother and thought to herself, *Yes, this is hard, watching Mama's dementia grow day by day as her body becomes more and more feeble. Moving her in with us has been difficult. Indeed there has been a price to pay. But having Mama tell Amy all the stories so she'll know about her history, well, it's the best investment I ever made.*

Lost and Found

I know you're going to think I'm being a smart aleck, but I like my mother much better now that she has lost her mind! When I was little, she was a really boring, bland person. Everything about her life and ours was routine. Take Fridays, for example. Every Friday we had fish (Mrs. Paul's® Fish Sticks, to be exact), macaroni and cheese (Kraft®) and cole slaw (made with Marzetti® dressing). It is important that you note the Registered R because she never made anything from scratch. And it wasn't just Friday. Sunday after church was ham (and Monday and Tuesday packed lunches were ham and cheese sandwiches). Sunday evening was bar-be-que beef sandwiches (ok Manwich®) and the rest of the cole slaw. Monday was Swiss steak, Tuesday was meatloaf (and Wednesday and Thursdays packed lunches were______, yep meatloaf), Wednesday was chicken and dumplings, and Thursday was liver and onions (yuck!). Saturdays we were on our own to eat leftovers (I think because my Dad spent the day at the club, playing golf, then having my mother join him for dinner and then play cards with other couples).

Everything was like that. You didn't even have to look at the calendar to know what day it was! She washed on Monday, ironed on Tuesday, volunteered in the library at our school on Wednesday, got her hair washed and set on Thursday, cleaned the house on Friday, worked in the garden on Saturday and went to church on Sunday.

I don't ever remember her really laughing out loud, raising her voice in anger, being sad and crying, or doing anything on the spur of the moment.

But now she is much older - 71, to be exact - and she has Alzheimer's. Most of the time she doesn't recognize me, but she is always glad to see me and she is a hoot. I never know what she's going to be wearing, what crazy activities she'll be doing, or who she will be pretending to be. She really reminds me of a very precocious, imaginative child. I look forward to every visit. I go every Monday, Wednesday, and Friday for sure (ok, so I'm my mother's daughter).

A couple of months ago, I walked into her room and there she was, hanging onto her walker, swinging her hips, tapping her toe and singing up a storm, accompanying her Benny Goodman record. As soon as she saw me, she insisted that I dance with her and kept begging, excitedly, over and over, "Dip me! Dip me!"

"I wish Daddy would come and dance with me," she said. (She always called my father Daddy. I only learned his real name when I was old enough to read whom the mail was addressed to.)

"Did Daddy like to dance?" I asked her.

"Oh, no!" she exclaimed. "That would have been too much excitement for him!"

I was concerned that all this dancing was too much excitement for her, so I put on another one of her favorite records, but one that had a slower pace, and sat her down in her favorite chair. I tried each time I visited to get her to exercise her mind and pull out things she remembered. I always brought a little tape recorder with me because I wanted to have these times, especially the lucid moments, to listen to after she was gone.

This visit I not only got stories, I finally found my real mother!

"You know," she said, "I loved Daddy so much. I tried very hard to be just what he wanted me to be. He was a very smart man. And so organized. Why, he had a place for everything and everything had its place."

Boy, did I remember that! Once I had snooped in their chest of drawers, looking for hidden Christmas presents, and found that he had all his socks in line, according to color. Then when I looked in the closet, I saw all the white shirts, lined up on hangers, facing the same way, all the suits in a row - one black, two gray and two navy. But that wasn't the best. The best was his workroom in the basement. All the tools were hung up on the pegboard and each tool had a black outline around it, so you knew that's where it went.

"Daddy didn't like surprises either," she whispered, as though it was some deep, dark secret. "He said surprises meant that things weren't under control."

Whoa, wait a minute. Was my mother's routine, day in and day out, year after year, done to keep my father happy?

"Didn't Daddy ever want to do something, well, spontaneous?" I asked. "Like maybe not having fish sticks on Friday?"

"Oh my, no!" she gasped, wide-eyed. "Why Fridays were always fish sticks and macaroni and cheese and cole slaw. Sunday it was ham at noon, bar-be-ques for supper. Monday was Swiss steak, Tuesday was meatloaf, Wednesday was chicken and dumplings and Thursday was liver and onions."

She shuddered when she recalled the liver and onions and whispered even more softly, "I hate liver and onions."

"Oh and every Saturday I would dress up and meet Daddy at the club for dinner and then we'd play cards with his men friends and their wives."

"Well, Mom, I know today is

only Wednesday, but let's get you dressed up and go out to eat," I suggested. "What would you like to eat?"

"I don't want chicken and dumplings!" she burst out, sounding almost like a child who was working up to a tantrum. "I absolutely don't want them!"

"Mom, you can have anything you want. What do you want?"

"I want pizza and a chocolate shake and I want them made from scratch," she declared, triumphantly.

I couldn't help it. I laughed out loud. Most people feel such a sense of loss when a parent gets Alzheimer's. Me? I think I've just found my real mother! And I really like the one I've found!

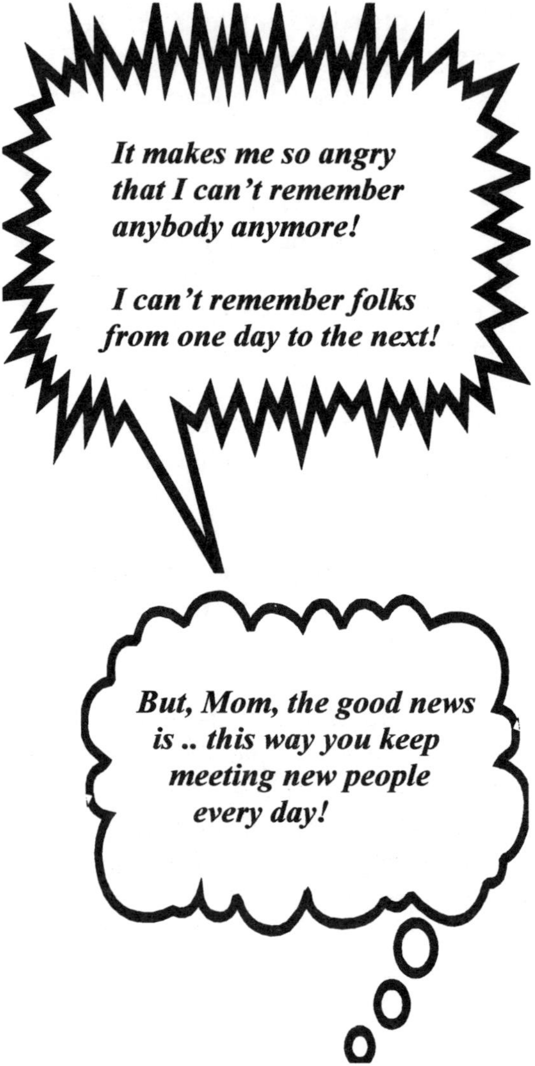
It makes me so angry that I can't remember anybody anymore!
I can't remember folks from one day to the next!
But, Mom, the good news is .. this way you keep meeting new people every day!

Mother Always Liked You Best!

"Sis, I just can't take it anymore! She really hates me. All she ever does is criticize everything I do. Nothing suits her. She's mean and cranky and is making my life miserable. If you don't take her to live with you, I'll wind up hating her. Please."

"How can I? Where would we put her? It's not fair to Tom to bring his mother-in-law here. And I don't think she'd be able to handle the kids' noise and everything. Anyway, you know mother always liked you best."

"She doesn't like me best. You're the one she always talks about it. You're the 'pretty one', the 'smart one', the one who gave her grandchildren. I am the single one, the one with no family of my own. That makes me the one to have to take care of her, right? Well, it's not fair to me either. I've been doing it for eight years. Now it's your turn."

"Sis, I just can't take it anymore! She really hates me. All she ever does is criticize everything I do. Nothing suits her. She's mean and cranky and is making our lives miserable. What are we going to do?"

"I can't take her back. Remember, I moved into this small apartment and I'm traveling for work. You know she really did always like you best. She doesn't hate you. I just can't take her back."

"Then we're going to have to put her in a nursing home. We looked into it and it's really expensive. We've got the kids' braces and Tom's student loans to repay. Can you do it? After all, she really did like you best."

"No, I can't afford it. No, she didn't like me best. No, I will not take her back. You've got her. You figure out what to do with her."

"Sis, how can you be so mean? She's our mother! Fine, we'll keep her here. You know, maybe she didn't like you best after all."

Throwaway Mama

Throwaway Mama sitting in her room
No one comes to see her
No one sees her tears
No one there to hug her
No one knows her fears

Throwaway Mama sitting in her room
Listening for her kids
Listening for the phone to ring
Listening for her friends
Listening for her heart to sing

Throwaway Mama sitting in her room
Waiting for her bath
Waiting for the hours to go by
Waiting for her meal
Waiting for her time to die

Throwaway Mama sitting in her room
Angels keep watch over her
Angels weep and sigh
Angels try to comfort her
Angels want to know why

Throwaway Mama?

The Wooden Bowl

A frail old woman went to live with her son, daughter-in-law and four year old granddaughter. The old woman's hands trembled, her eyesight was blurred and her step faltered. Every evening the family ate together, but the elderly mother's shaky hands and failing eyesight made eating difficult. Peas rolled off her spoon onto the floor. When she tried to pick up her glass, liquid spilled all over the tablecloth.

The son and daughter-in-law became fed up with the spills, the food on the floor and the sight of this messy eating. So they wouldn't have to watch this every night at the table, they set up a small table in the corner with a large plastic sheet under it. There, every evening, the mother ate alone. Because she had broken several pieces of the china when they slipped from her hands, they put her food in a wooden bowl. Every once in awhile they would look in her direction and noticed, as she fumbled to eat, that she had tears in her eyes. The couple's anger would flair whenever she spilled something and they would admonish her to be more careful.

Her granddaughter watched it all in silence. One evening before dinner, the father noticed his daughter, sitting on the floor, playing with wood scraps and asked what she was doing.

"Oh. I am making a little bowl for you and Mama to eat your food out of when I grow up."

Author Unknown

A Day in the Life of a Woman – Wife, Mother, Career Woman, Caregiver

5:30 a.m. Wake up, get out of bed, do a few stretching and bending exercises, find my glasses.

5:45 a.m. Help mother get out of bed, go to bathroom and get settled at a table in her room; then go to kitchen, fix her tea and a glass of juice.

6:10 a.m. Wake up the kids (a couple of times), pick up clothes and check to be sure all homework is in backpacks, while I'm doing it.

6:15 a.m. Fix kids breakfast, grab a cup of coffee and empty dishwasher.

6:25 a.m. Take a cup of coffee to my husband. Brush my teeth, wash my face, dress and put on make-up while the kids are eating (and shout downstairs to ask my husband to get them to stop picking on each other!) Oh, and make the beds!

6:45 a.m. Go back to mother's room, clear away breakfast dishes, get her settled in her chair by the TV. Check to make sure she has everything she needs on her table next to the chair.

6:50 a.m. Back to kitchen to get kids to finish up, get their backpacks and walk up to the school bus.

6:55 a.m. Fix a bowl of cereal for myself, eat standing up at the counter while I quickly read the morning paper and go over the day's schedules with my husband (like who is taking the kids to soccer practice, when everyone will be home for dinner, and which meetings each of us has).

7:00 a.m. Mother's caregiver arrives. I pick up the kitchen, make a whirlwind inspection through the first floor to get any glasses, plates, etc.; then go to my office and put papers in my briefcase, stop to say goodbye to Mother and leave.

7:20 a.m. Leave house and am in the car for 40 minutes during which time I leave four voice mail messages (on my hands-free mobile phone), record on my voice-activated tape recorder things I need to remember to do and buy and thoughts relevant to client activities.

8:00 a.m. - noon Meetings with two different clients, using travel time to make phone calls, stop at dry cleaners and get gas.

Noon Meet with group from a non-profit for lunch

1:15 p.m. Leave parking lot to get to 2:00 appointment with time to pick up prescription for mother.

2:00 p.m. Meeting with client

3:00 p.m. Drive home with time in car spent on phone calls.

3:20 p.m. Arrive home, check on mother and the caregiver, pick up soccer equipment the kids forgot. Dash to school.

3:30 p.m. Arrive at school, pick up kids and take them to practice.

3:45 p.m. Leave soccer field and drive to post office to mail packages.

4:15 p.m. Finally get through line at post office. Drive back to soccer field.

4:25 p.m. Arrive at soccer field, sit in car, check voice mail, make calls.

4:35 p.m. Kids pile into car, drop off several and head home.

5:00 p.m. Reach home. Caregiver leaves. Get dinner for Mom and sit and chat a few minutes while she is eating.

5:20 p.m. Leave Mom while she is eating and go start dinner for kids.

5:45 p.m. While kids are eating, clean up Mom's dinner dishes, start a load of laundry.

6:05 p.m. Sit with kids and talk about their day and homework they need help with.

6:30 p.m. Kids clean up kitchen; I go and start second load of laundry

6:40 p.m. Kids visit with Gram, I do grocery list, catch the end of the news, and quickly read the evening paper.

7:00 p.m. Daughter needs supplies for school project, so we run to the store.

7:55 p.m. Back home. Look in on Mother, help her to bathroom, get her settled back in chair; put second load in dryer, fold first load. Kids are doing homework. Stop to help with hard problems.

8:35 p.m. Husband arrives home. Reheat dinner for him. Sit and chat with him, while he's eating.

9:00 p.m. Fold second load of laundry and put baskets by the stairs. Take Mother's to her and put it away. Then go upstairs and put ours away.

9:20 p.m. Telephone call. A meeting time has been changed. There are four people on my list I have to notify.

9:40 p.m. Help Mother bathe and get ready for bed. Get her into bed and turn on TV so she can watch 10 p.m. news.

10:00 p.m. Start urging kids to finish up with whatever they are doing and get baths. This goes on for at least 30 minutes! In between I pop up and down on the couch, trying to watch the news with my husband.

10:30 p.m. Check on Mother. Start in earnest to get kids to bed.

11:00 p.m. Finally! Everyone's in bed. Go to computer and start on client assignment.

12:30 a.m. Turn off computer. Put coffee on timer. Check on everyone. Take shower and go to bed.

12:50 a.m. My husband is already asleep, so I read until I fall asleep.

I Watch My Mother

I watch my sister-in-law closely. She is pregnant - heavy and cumbersome with her third child. She has a daughter almost three and a son almost eighteen months. She is consumed with diapers, feedings, playtime and naptime. She has little time for herself but she seems to thrive on her self-imposed regimen.

I watch my mother closely. (She is not pregnant.) She has no children at home. She has no buses to meet, no blue jeans to hem, no new projects to oversee. Her grandchildren have parents who are fully capable of running their own lives (most of the time) and meeting their own children's needs.

My sister-in-law, even if she so chooses, has little time to pursue hobbies, interests and outside pursuits. My mother, on the other hand, has the time to widen her horizons, expand her boundaries and develop skills and talents too long ignored under the guise of being a hands-on mother and grandmother.

My mother's role is changing. Her eldest daughter's children are becoming self-sufficient and her youngest daughter, with her husband and children, is moving away. Her only son has his own life, his own priorities.

"I use to have a knot in my stomach everyday around 3 PM," one of my older acquaintances once told me, "because I knew in minutes my kids would come bursting through the door - home from school - breaking the peaceful solitude of my day. NOW I have a pit in my stomach every day around 3 PM because I know NO children will be bursting through my door at 3 PM - they are grown and gone."

I watch my mother closely. She talks of not being needed. She infers she is being shut out. I respond as best I can - reassuring her that it is not a case of not being needed, but rather a natural pulling away that all offspring do in order to assert their independence - and make their own way.

I watch my mother closely. She seems to be listening. She discusses plans to run an institutional gift shop. She plays cards spontaneously with friends and goes on a day's outing to Indianapolis on a whim. But still she grieves.

A holiday weekend comes. My brother is busy with his new wife and her family. I am booked for an extended family outing with my husband's relatives. My sister and her brood are occupied with packing for their move to Virginia. My mother and father are alone.

We go to the park and toss Frisbees. An elderly couple approaches me hesitantly - asking if I would take a picture of them picnicking on a blanket amidst the spring bulbs and read-to-bloom trees. I do it eagerly - hungry for their story.

"It's for our daughter, who lives in Milwaukee," they explain. "We want to show her we have a life." They laugh and so do I.

By 5 PM, we are home. The kids are still wound up so they help their father mow the lawn. They help me weed. In between chores, they play soccer and toss baseballs in the back yard where I work. I am surrounded by them and their activities - temporarily safe in a cocoon of my own weaving.

My mother and father are alone.

At 7:30 PM the phone rings. I answer hurriedly. It's hard to hear. Louie is practicing his sax five feet away and Sam and Max are fighting over the TV.

It's my mother - a note of jubilation in her voice. "Guess where we went?" she asks gleefully.

"I can't imagine," I reply honestly.

"To the zoo," she exclaims. "We went to the zoo. Just your father and I. And, oh, what a time we had!"

"Good for her," I think. I am delighted for them. And I silently pray that they will have many years of good health – these years without children. I want to cherish these years when they could "do for themselves" because I know that the time will come when my brother, sister and I will once again become parents - parenting our parents.

Perhaps there will come a day when I will be bundling her up and taking her to the zoo. Even then I will watch my mother.

by Iris Ruth Pastor

I never envisioned taking on the role Mom had taken on with my grandparents. Both her mother and my father's father lived with us from the time I was twelve until I was twenty-one. Actually my role was different. Mom didn't work outside the home. She devoted her life to taking care of all of us.

I, on the other hand, had never even been a full time parent! I had always worked. I had raised my kids to be self-sufficient. When Mom moved in with us, I wanted to work out ways Mom could remain self-sufficient, also. Before and after work, I did all the things she couldn't do and she did the things she could. As time went on, she needed my help more and more and was able to do less and less on her own. To everyone else, it looked as though we were handling everything just fine. However, I was becoming overwhelmed with the responsibility and I just couldn't seem to get it into words.

It all came to a head that Christmas I was recovering from the fall. With hand in cast, bruises all over my body and aches and pains everywhere, I didn't have enough energy to get myself up and going each day, let alone help Mom. So I did what any creative, Type A would do. I ran away from home! With a trashy novel, bottle of wine and flannel gown and thermal socks, I checked into a local hotel on Christmas Eve and stayed there, tucked under the covers, until the day after Christmas!

When I returned home, everyone in the family was still in shock from my behavior, but it accomplished what I had been unable to do -- get us communicating about doing what was best for Mom -- and for me.

The results were a flurry of winter activities. We totally revamped the house, widening doorways, re-installing fixtures and appliances so she could reach them in her wheelchair, and having trained caregivers come in several times a week to help out. We got her a new wheelchair that was easier to get around in and a great lift/recliner chair that she had to fight off the grandchildren to get into! She had her Lifeline monitor so, if I wasn't right there, she could call for assistance from our community paramedics and police.

I made some adjustments, too. I converted the lower level of the house to an office and started doing my work from home. It was strange at first. I had never been a home-based business and now I was sharing my home with associates and clients, care givers and support people. When the phone rang, I had a heck of a time figuring out if it was my home phone, my mother's or the kids', the office line or the FAX! It drove me crazy. I didn't want to reach out and touch someone, I wanted to rip phone lines out of the wall!

My approach to PATIENCE used to be like the cartoon I had on the bulletin board. The woman is looking up toward the heavens and she is praying, "Lord give me patience, and I want it NOW!" Mom's attitude was pretty much the same. We both always expected things to happen when we wanted. Neither of us ever thought that when we asked for a chore to be done, we would have to state that we wanted it done NOW. Now was the time we had asked, now was the time we wanted it done.

What I learned was that time stretches out even more for a person when they are confined. It drove Mom crazy when she would ask for something to be done and it didn't happen immediately. Lots of times it didn't happen because on my *Scale of One To Ten* prioritization list, it had slipped to #7. And then, quite honestly, I would forget. Then I'd get the "gotcha line." Do you know what those are? Those are the statements people make that push your buttons. Mom's would be, "I know how busy you are, but when you have time, would you...?" Or even better, when my brother and his wife would come from out of town for a visit, she would have a whole list of things for them to do because "she hasn't gotten around to it yet." The she, of course, meaning me.

Now it made absolutely no difference how she actually meant those statements. For me it launched the guilt and defensive modes, guilt for not doing what she asked, when she asked, and defensive because I didn't want my brother to think I was neglecting her. So, most of the time I hustled to it.

Were the things she wanted important? Well, yes and no. Important to her because she had to look at the cobwebs in the corner. (My thought on cobwebs is that you should spray paint them and strategically place silk flowers for an avant-garde accent piece.) She also had Gertrude and needed to have her changed regularly. Gertrude was her concrete goose on her screened in porch. When Mom was able, she made all kinds of outfits for her - one for every season, every holiday. She even had outfits to cheer on our sports teams.

My job - dress Gertrude. No big deal, right? Well, no, but irritating for Mom, I'm sure, when Gertrude was out on the porch, freezing her little concrete tush off in a festive holiday frock, when she should be wrapped in her faux fur coat and hat. (And, ok, she was still dressed in her Halloween witches outfit at Thanksgiving, but I got her into her pilgrim garb on Turkey Day in time for the last chorus of "We gather together..." and the first course of dinner.)

Over time, we have both learned a new kind of patience, one that wasn't instantaneous, that's for sure, but one which recognized that some things were more important than others. Many of our habits were from another time and had no place in the lives we were sharing. Of course, we'd get out of sorts with each other, but we'd get over it and get on with it. And, if that didn't work, I could always call my brother and lament, "Guess what <u>your</u> mother did today."

A Caregiver's Bill of Rights

I have the right

to take care of myself. This is not an act of selfishness. It will give me the capability of taking better care of my parent(s).

to seek help from others even though my parent(s) may object. I recognize the limits of my own endurance and strength.

to maintain facets of my own life that do not include the parent(s) I care for. I know that I do everything that I reasonably can for them, and I have the right to do some things just for myself.

to get angry, depressed, and express other difficult feelings occasionally.

to reject any attempt by my parent(s) (either conscious or unconscious) to manipulate me through guilt, anger, or depression.

to receive consideration, affection, forgiveness, and acceptance for what I do from my parent(s) for as long as I offer these qualities in return.

to take pride in what I am accomplishing and to applaud the courage it has sometimes taken to meet the needs of my parent(s).

to protect my individuality and my right to make a life for myself that will sustain me when the time comes that I no longer am the caregiver for my parent(s).

From

Caregiving: Helping An Aging Loved One

Jo Horne

STRIVE

Here's my list of things you need as you strive to become the best caregiver you can be…

S Support systems, professional and personal

T Time – to spend with your elders, your family, your friends, yourself

R Relatives who care for you and with whom you are not too proud to ask for help when you need it

I Insurance – not only health, but long-term care, stewardship annuities – protection you should have for your elders and for you

V Very good friends who will give you a hand to help, their hearts in understanding, a shoulder to cry on, and a link to life beyond caregiving

E Energy to stay the course and survive the caregiving experience!

"If I hear that damned little bell one more time, I'm going to take it and..." Marsha stopped mid-sentence because her little girl was looking at her with really big eyes. Marsha hardly ever swore but her mother was driving her crazy! She could no longer get out of her bed and anytime she wanted something she rang her bell. And just like Pavlov's little dog, Marsha went running to see what she wanted.

At the beginning Marsha had run willingly. But lately her mother didn't really need anything. She just made up excuses to get Marsha to come into her room. And when Marsha did, they always seemed to wind up yelling at each other, a combination of her mother's failed hearing and Marsha's frustration. Mostly, they argued over the little things – the way her mother would throw things on the floor instead of putting them on the bedside table, would spill her water glass everywhere because she didn't watch what she was doing, or turn her TV so loud it could be heard even outside the house.

"Mother, I'll be there in a minute," she yelled. "I'm trying to get this chewing gum out of Audrey's hair.

"Now sit still, so I can get it out," she ordered her daughter. "How in the world did you ever make such a mess? When I am done here, you are going to get a time out in your room to think about being more careful."

The child look at her mother. "Mama, I won't have to stay there always like Grammy, will I?"

"Oh, honey, no," Marsha said, hugging her child.

"That's good," Audrey replied. "I don't want a damned little bell."

Kidnapping Mama

When Sarah's father died, her mother became part of the furniture. Sadie occupied the chaise lounge in Sarah's solarium and ceased to function. She only ate when Sarah prepared food for her and only interacted with the family when they physically pulled her into the activity.

Finally, after six months, Sarah couldn't stand it any longer. She decided to take her vacation days, leave her husband and children to hold the fort, and just put her mother in the car and start driving.

When she shared this idea with her mother, Sadie was adamant. She had no intention of going.

"Your father and I traveled already," she said. "There's nothing left that I want to see."

"Oh, Mama, this will be fun and it will be good for you," Sarah shot back. "Beside it will give us a chance to spend some time together, just the two of us."

So, she packed the car, filled the tank with gas and asked her mother if she wanted to go for a ride to the store with her.

"All right," Sadie said. "As long as we're back in time for me to see my shows."

Sadie reluctantly got her purse, stuffed it with Kleenex, fumbled to get her sweater on and ever so slowly maneuvered out the door with her walker. She looked for all the world like a moody heifer being prodded along!

Sarah's heart pounded as she passed the shopping mall and entered the highway. My God, she thought, I'm kidnapping Mama!

Just like a small child, Sadie always dozed off when she was in the car. She woke up when the car came to a stop and Sarah had turned off the ignition. "This isn't the store," she cried. "What have you done, gotten us lost?"

"No, Mama, I think we're going to find something," Sarah replied

"What?" Sadie asked, sighing with absolute frustration. She didn't like it when she didn't know what was going on and that seemed to be happening more and more frequently.

"Mama, things are changing," Sarah said softly, tears running down her face. "You've said it yourself. You've got body rot! I know you try to be funny about it, but I want to spend time with you, while you remember who I am."

"Ok, Sarah, I'll do this for you," Sadie sighed.

Sarah smiled to herself. Of all the talents her mother had, the one for which she could have won the Oscar or Tony or Emmy was her sigh. She perfected the sigh into a whole language – relief, anger, disappointment, vexation, tiredness, sadness, frustration, boredom, disgust, pain, grief, reluctant acceptance, utter resignation, you name it. It was an amazing skill. One sigh was a whole soliloquy or the briefest, *bon mot*.

"Come on, Mama, this will be fun," she cajoled. "We're in Nashville."

"Oh, can we go to the Grand Ole Opry?" Sadie sounded just like an excited child. "You know how I love my Country music."

"Mama, we're going to see it all," Sarah answered. "And after we spend a couple of days here we're going on to see the love of your life!"

"Phooey, we can't do that. He's been dead for a long time. But he lives right here," she said, pointing to her heart. Sadie smiled and started humming ***Love Me Tender***.

"Come on, Mama, where have you always wanted to go?"

"Oh, you mean Graceland?" Sadie sat up and stared at her daughter. "Really, Sarah, really? Are we going to Graceland? Your father would <u>not</u> take me there and I always said it was the one place I had to go before I die. Oh my, I'm finally going to see it!

"Oh, Sarah, thank you. You know, I was really angry with you when I first woke up from dozing here in the car.

I felt like you had kidnapped me! I'm so glad you did! Body rot or not, here I come, Elvis, here I come."

----Original Message----

From: Elsie [elsie@aol.com]

Sent: Thursday, June 27 11:31 PM

To: sis@aol.com

Subject: I wish I could remember just the good times!

Hi - Mom's been gone three years today and, even after all this time, I can't believe how much I still think about the really bad times, especially when she was really mean and nasty to me and the kids. It still hurts -- some of the things she said and called me. You'd think I'd grow up and get a life, huh?

Elsie

----Reply----

No, we all know that the ones who can hurt us the most are the ones we love the most and who, when all is said and done, love us the most. It's one of those anomalies of life. Our parents can be at the heart of some of our best times and at the soul of our worst. It's a struggle, but the only way to really have a life of our own is to try to remember the times they touched our heart, not broke it.

Mom could be a real, pardon the expression and I know I am talking about our mother, bitch when she wanted to and she didn't have to put much effort into it! But then again, she could be a really great person to be around for the kids, and us again without trying. I suspect our own children can pretty much say the same about us. As much as we say we will not be like our parents, we can't help ourselves. It's like the day we look in the mirror and see the resemblance and hear mother's voice coming out of our mouths that we realize it all comes with the territory.

I think it is our place in life to try to be more at the heart of the best times than at the soul of the worst. It's a struggle a lot of the time, but we have to keep trying. I think more than previous generations, we are able to look at our parents as human beings and accept their flaws rather than in times past when they had that layer of "respect" that would not allow their children to admit that they saw them as less than perfect. I guess I have learned that I don't have to have liked what our parents did or the way they were to love them. That's one of those “comes around things.” How many times did we have to remember to tell our kids "I don't like what you are doing, but I still love you"? I've found it's the same later in life with parents.

Ah, I wax philosophical. It's not about "growing up and getting a life". It's about admitting there were the hurts and trying to work on remembering the good times. The hurts run deep, but the good times, once they have a chance to surface, float a whole lot better since they are lighter. Don't beat your self up, especially when you were doing a good thing. You took care of her for a long time. And then it was our turn. We got it, too. Let's just hope we don't give our kids the grief and aggravation she gave us! On second thought... never mind.

Love,

Sis

Ready To Go

For the last couple years of Mama's life, she made it very clear to all of us that she was ready to go. The quality of her life was slipping and, as she often pointed out to me, she had lived a full, wonderful life and this current life she found herself living didn't hold a candle to the past life she had enjoyed. She laughingly would say that she had been there, done that and had a whole chest full of T-shirts with sayings that captured the adventure or emotion of the moment.

At first it bothered me that she felt this way. She seemed so eager to leave us? Were her words digs on the caregiving she was receiving? Didn't she care about how we felt about losing her? Didn't we matter anymore? How would I ever get along without her? Sixty years is a long time to know someone and then say goodbye.

"Mama, how can you want to leave me?" I cried. "You make me feel like I haven't been a good daughter."

"No, you haven't been a good daughter," she retorted. "You've been a great daughter, but you'll know, too, when you get old, when it is time to go."

Then, as we talked honestly about her thoughts and feelings, I realized that she truly felt that this life had come to completion and that it was time to move on to the life she had been promised ever since her earliest childhood Sunday school classes. She had no fear of dying. Others were waiting for her – her husband, her sister, her brother-in-law, her parents, and grandparents and so many friends...

"You know, I figure I have lived almost 30,000 days and I have to tell you, there has been more laughter than tears," she said.

That's my Mama. She always said there were two basic emotional expressions - laughter and tears.

Yes, there were tears when she died. But she was ready to go. Now I think of her most at the moments of laughter. Her laugh rings in my ears. At this precise moment, she and I share that love again that began at my birth and will continue, even when she and I meet again.

And I thank her for the greatest gift she gave me, laughter.

As she always said,
"She who laughs, lasts."

Judy Pettigrew was the primary caregiver for her mother for eighteen years (with "time off" for good behavior every once in awhile). At the same time, as a single parent, she raised two children (and actually got them to 21 alive) and fed three cats (who preferred she not smother them with attention), founded and built three businesses (and mothered them just the way she did her kids), was involved in many organizations (she's *just a gal who can't say no*), kept up a house (well, sometimes!), and survived it all with her sense of humor in tact.

Judy has entertained and enlightened audiences all over the U.S. with her presentation of ***Sending Mama To Her Room***.

She is available for speaking engagements, corporate work/life programs and personal development workshops. She can be reached at:

WOW! Unlimited Inc.

888-URA WOW 1
(888-872-9691)

or
mom@wowunlimited.com